Meralgia Paresthetica

A Beginner's Quick Start Guide to Managing the Condition Through Diet and Other Home Remedies, with Sample Curated Recipes

mf

copyright © 2022 Patrick Marshwell

All rights reserved No part of this book may be reproduced, or stored in a retrieval system, or transmitted in any form or by any means, electronic, mechanical, photocopying, recording, or otherwise, without express written permission of the publisher.

Disclaimer

By reading this disclaimer, you are accepting the terms of the disclaimer in full. If you disagree with this disclaimer, please do not read the guide.

All of the content within this guide is provided for informational and educational purposes only, and should not be accepted as independent medical or other professional advice. The author is not a doctor, physician, nurse, mental health provider, or registered nutritionist/dietician. Therefore, using and reading this guide does not establish any form of a physician-patient relationship.

Always consult with a physician or another qualified health provider with any issues or questions you might have regarding any sort of medical condition. Do not ever disregard any qualified professional medical advice or delay seeking that advice because of anything you have read in this guide. The information in this guide is not intended to be any sort of medical advice and should not be used in lieu of any medical advice by a licensed and qualified medical professional.

The information in this guide has been compiled from a variety of known sources. However, the author cannot attest to or guarantee the accuracy of each source and thus should not be held liable for any errors or omissions.

You acknowledge that the publisher of this guide will not be held liable for any loss or damage of any kind incurred as a result of this guide or the reliance on any information provided within this guide. You acknowledge and agree that you assume all risk and responsibility for any action you undertake in response to the information in this guide.

Using this guide does not guarantee any particular result (e.g., weight loss or a cure). By reading this guide, you acknowledge that there are no guarantees to any specific outcome or results you can expect.

All product names, diet plans, or names used in this guide are for identification purposes only and are the property of their respective owners. The use of these names does not imply endorsement. All other trademarks cited herein are the property of their respective owners.

Where applicable, this guide is not intended to be a substitute for the original work of this diet plan and is, at most, a supplement to the original work for this diet plan and never a direct substitute. This guide is a personal expression of the facts of that diet plan.

Where applicable, persons shown in the cover images are stock photography models and the publisher has obtained the rights to use the images through license agreements with third-party stock image companies.

Table of Contents

Introduction	7
What Is Meralgia Paresthetica?	9
What causes meralgia paresthetica?	9
What are the symptoms of meralgia paresthetica?	11
Who is at risk of getting meralgia paresthetica?	12
How is meralgia paresthetica diagnosed?	13
What are the medical treatments for meralgia paresthetica?	14
What are the complications of meralgia paresthetica?	15
How to prevent meralgia paresthetica?	16
Managing Meralgia Paresthetica through Natural Methods	18
Managing Meralgia Paresthetica through Diet	22
Principles of Meralgia Paresthetica Diet	22
Benefits of a Meralgia Paresthetica Diet	24
Disadvantages of The Meralgia Paresthetica Diet	27
5-Step-by-Step Guide on How to Get Started with Meralgia Paresthetica Diet	29
Step 1: Consult Your Healthcare Provider	29
Step 2: Incorporate Anti-Inflammatory Foods	30
Step 3: Boost Omega-3 Fatty Acids	32
Step 4: Eliminate Processed and Sugary Foods	35
Step 5: Stay Hydrated and Track Your Progress	38
Foods to Eat	42
Foods to Avoid	44
7-Day Sample Meal Plan for Meralgia Paresthetica	46
Sample Recipes	49
Baked Flounder	50
Asian-Themed Macrobiotic Bowl	51
Chicken Salad	53
Baked Salmon	55

Asian Zucchini Salad	57
Low FODMAP Burger	59
Asparagus and Greens Salad with Tahini and Poppy Seed Dressing	61
Stir-Fried Cabbage and Apples	63
Roasted Chicken Thighs	64
Arugula and Mushroom Salad	65
Fresh Asparagus Salad	67
Tuna Salad	69
Roasted Veggies	70
Roasted Pumpkin and Brussels Sprouts	72
Quinoa Stuffed Peppers	73
Conclusion	**75**
FAQs	**79**
References and Helpful Links	**82**

Introduction

A large nerve that travels from the lower back to the legs is called the femoral nerve. It gives the front and center of the thigh, as well as much of the lower leg and foot, the ability to feel and move. The sensation of touch is carried to the skin on the outside aspect of the thigh by a branch of the femoral nerve known as the lateral femoral cutaneous nerve (LFCN). The LFCN descends from the upper buttock, through the hip, and into the thigh, beginning at the posterior aspect of the thigh.

Meralgia paresthetica, also known as Bernhardt-Roth syndrome, is a condition in which the lateral femoral cutaneous nerve is damaged or put under too much pressure, resulting in numbness, pain, or a burning sensation on the outer thigh. This condition can also be referred to as the Bernhardt-Roth syndrome.

The majority of the time, meralgia paresthetica may be addressed with straightforward adjustments to one's lifestyle, such as switching to clothes with a looser fit. On the other hand, medicine or surgery could be necessary for certain patients who have more severe cases of meralgia paresthetica. If you are having any of these symptoms, you need to make an appointment with a medical professional as soon as possible so that they can recommend the therapy that will be most effective for you.

In this beginner's start guide, we'll cover the following topics:

- What causes meralgia paresthetica?
- What are the symptoms of meralgia paresthetica?
- Who is at risk of getting meralgia paresthetica?
- How is meralgia paresthetica diagnosed?
- What are the medical treatments for meralgia paresthetica?
- How to prevent meralgia paresthetica?
- How to manage meralgia paresthetica through natural methods?
- How to manage meralgia paresthetica through diet?

As you read this guide, we hope that you will find the material to be useful in comprehending what meralgia paresthetica is, its causes and risk factors, as well as how the illness may be managed by nutrition, and that you will also find out how to treat the condition with diet.

What Is Meralgia Paresthetica?

Meralgia Paresthetica, also known as lateral femoral cutaneous neuropathy, refers to a condition characterized by the compression or irritation of the lateral femoral cutaneous nerve. This nerve is responsible for providing sensation to the outer thigh, and when affected, it can lead to various sensory disturbances in this region.

Although often not serious, Meralgia Paresthetica can result in discomfort that may impact daily activities, making it important to understand and manage effectively with appropriate medical care and lifestyle adjustments.

What causes meralgia paresthetica?

Meralgia paresthetica is almost often brought on by constricted garments or belts that impose pressure on the lateral femoral cutaneous nerve. This is the most prevalent cause of the condition. This is something that can occur if you wear pants that are too tight, belts, or any other type of clothing that creates pressure on your waist or thighs. Meralgia paresthetica can also be caused by other factors, such as:

- ***Obesity***: Meralgia paresthetica is a condition that can be caused by carrying additional weight, which puts pressure on the lateral femoral cutaneous nerve. If you are overweight and suffer from thigh discomfort, numbness, or tingling, you should discuss the possibility of meralgia paresthetica with your primary care physician.
- ***Pregnancy***: Meralgia paresthetica is a condition that is frequently brought on by pregnancy. This is because the expanding uterus and the additional weight might exert strain on the lateral femoral cutaneous nerve.
- ***Diabetes***: Diabetes patients have an increased likelihood of developing meralgia paresthetica because high blood sugar levels can be damaging to nerves. Damage to the nerve that extends from the abdomen down into the leg might be the root cause of this ailment, which manifests itself as a burning, tingling, or numbing sensation in the affected thigh. It is common for this nerve to get injured in diabetic patients as a result of high blood sugar levels.
- ***Herniated disc***: The symptoms of meralgia paresthetica can be brought on by a herniated disc in the lower back, which puts pressure on the lateral femoral cutaneous nerve.
- ***Surgery***: Meralgia paresthetica can be caused by injury to the lateral femoral cutaneous nerve, which can occur if surgery is performed on the hip, thigh, or abdomen.

- *Trauma*: Meralgia paresthetica can be caused by a damaged lateral femoral cutaneous nerve, which can be caused by an injury to the hip, thigh, or abdomen.

If you have any of these risk factors, you should discuss the likelihood of meralgia paresthetica with your primary care physician as soon as possible. The problem must be diagnosed and treated promptly to be managed effectively.

What are the symptoms of meralgia paresthetica?

A burning feeling on the outer thigh is the symptom of meralgia paresthetica that is experienced by the vast majority of patients. Among the other symptoms are:

- *Numbness on the outer thigh*: You may feel like your thigh is "falling asleep."
- *Tingling on the outer thigh*: You may feel a pins-and-needles sensation on your outer thigh.
- *Pain on the outer thigh*: You may feel a sharp, burning pain on your outer thigh.
- *Weakness in the legs*: You may feel like your legs are weak or "rubbery."
- *Aching in the hip or groin*: You may feel a deep, aching pain in your hip or groin.

It is vital to consult a medical professional if you are having any of these symptoms, as they will be able to diagnose the origin of your condition and provide treatment suggestions.

Who is at risk of getting meralgia paresthetica?

Meralgia paresthetica affects women more frequently than it does males. Other potential dangers include the following:

- *Wearing tight-fitting clothing or belts*: Meralgia paresthetica is mostly brought on by the most prevalent cause, which is wearing belts or clothes that are too tight.
- *Obesity*: Carrying around excess weight due to obesity can exert strain on the lateral femoral cutaneous nerve, which can ultimately result in meralgia paresthetica.
- *Pregnancy*: Meralgia paresthetica can be caused by pregnancy because the additional weight that occurs with pregnancy can place pressure on the lateral femoral cutaneous nerve, which can then result in the condition.
- *Diabetes*: Because high blood sugar levels can be damaging to nerves, those who have diabetes have an increased likelihood of developing meralgia paresthetica.
- *Herniated disc*: A herniated disc in the lower back can induce meralgia paresthetica by putting pressure on the

lateral femoral cutaneous nerve and putting pressure on the nerve.
- *Surgery*: Operations on the hip, the thigh, or the abdomen can cause injury to the lateral femoral cutaneous nerve, which can result in meralgia paresthetica.
- *Trauma*: Meralgia paresthetica can be caused by trauma, namely an injury to the hip, thigh, or abdomen. This can injure the lateral femoral cutaneous nerve, which in turn causes the condition.

If you think you could be at risk for meralgia paresthetica, you should make an appointment with a medical professional as soon as possible so that they can diagnose the problem and advise you on how to treat it.

How is meralgia paresthetica diagnosed?

The condition known as meralgia paresthetica is often diagnosed through a combination of your symptoms and a physical examination. Your doctor will most likely inquire about your past medical history as well as the period in which you first noticed symptoms. In addition, he or she will carry out a physical examination, during which they will most likely apply pressure on or extend her thigh to determine whether or not doing so causes her to experience discomfort.

Your doctor may also prescribe further tests, such as an MRI or a nerve conduction study, to rule out the possibility of other illnesses in some instances.

- *MRI*: The magnetic resonance imaging (MRI) exam takes photographs of the inside of your body by using magnetic waves. Your doctor may be able to rule out other diseases, such as a herniated disc, with the use of this information.
- *Nerve conduction study*: An examination of nerve conduction, often known as a nerve conduction study, determines how efficiently electrical signals pass through your nerves. Your doctor may be able to eliminate additional illnesses, such as diabetes, using this information.

If you are suffering symptoms of meralgia paresthetica, you should make an appointment with a medical professional as soon as possible so that the illness may be correctly diagnosed and treated.

What are the medical treatments for meralgia paresthetica?

Avoiding garments or belts that are too tight-fitting is the therapy for meralgia paresthetica that is used most frequently. If you are overweight, decreasing weight can assist ease pressure on the lateral femoral cutaneous nerve. This is especially true for people who are obese.

The following are some more therapies for meralgia paresthetica:

- *Medications*: Your physician may recommend that you take medication to assist in easing symptoms. These drugs may include pain relievers, antidepressants, or anticonvulsants.
- *Injections*: To assist alleviate the pain, your doctor may choose to inject a local anesthetic or steroid drug into the affected region.
- *Surgery*: Surgery may be required in some circumstances to relieve the pressure that is being placed on the lateral femoral cutaneous nerve.

In most cases, these therapies are beneficial in reducing the discomfort associated with meralgia paresthetica. However, it is essential to make an appointment with a medical professional for them to accurately identify and treat the disease.

What are the complications of meralgia paresthetica?

The condition known as meralgia paresthetica is often a harmless one that does not result in any significant problems. However, the syndrome can, in extremely unusual circumstances, result in more significant complications such as the following:

- ***Chronic pain***: If the meralgia paresthetica condition is not addressed, it can lead to pain that does not go away.
- ***Nerve damage***: Meralgia paresthetica can, in extremely unusual situations, result in permanent damage to the nerves.

It is in your best interest to get medical care as soon as you have any symptoms related to meralgia paresthetica. This will allow the illness to be properly treated, and it will also help you prevent any problems that may arise as a result of the disease.

How to prevent meralgia paresthetica?

Wearing loose-fitting clothing and avoiding tight-fitting jeans, belts, and other items of clothing that impose pressure on your waist or thighs will help prevent the painful condition known as meralgia paresthetica. If you are overweight, lowering weight can help minimize your risk of meralgia paresthetica. This is especially true if you have a family history of the condition.

1. **Wear loose-fitting clothing**

    Wearing clothes that do not fit too closely is the most effective method for preventing meralgia paresthetica. Compression of the lateral femoral cutaneous nerve, which extends from the hip to the thigh, is the root cause of this disorder.

This nerve can be pinched if you wear belts or garments that are too tight, which can cause discomfort, numbness, and tingling in the thigh. If you are prone to meralgia paresthetica, you should avoid wearing belts and garments that are too tight on you at all costs.

2. **Lose weight if you are overweight**

Meralgia paresthetica is a condition that can be caused by carrying additional weight, which puts pressure on the lateral femoral cutaneous nerve. Weight loss can help reduce the symptoms of meralgia paresthetica and relieve the pressure that is being placed on the nerves.

Decreasing weight can help improve your general health and lessen the chance of acquiring various health disorders such as heart disease, diabetes, and arthritis. In addition, losing weight can help enhance your overall quality of life. If you are overweight, you should consult your physician about a weight loss program that is tailored to your specific needs.

By adhering to these straightforward recommendations, you may help prevent meralgia paresthetica and live a life free from discomfort. If you have any questions or concerns regarding this disease, you should make an appointment with your primary care physician as soon as possible.

Managing Meralgia Paresthetica through Natural Methods

Meralgia paresthetica is a disorder that has the potential to be both painful and frustrating. You are in luck since several natural remedies can assist you in taking care of your problems.

1. *Diet*: Consuming a diet high in nutrients is essential for the management of meralgia paresthetica. It is possible to lessen the severity of symptoms by avoiding items that are known to cause inflammation, such as processed meals, sweets, and unhealthy fats. Consuming foods that are known to lower inflammation, such as those rich in omega-3 fatty acids, may also be beneficial in this regard.

2. *Exercise*: Physical activity is an essential component in the management of meralgia paresthetica. Walking and swimming are examples of low-impact workouts that can help strengthen the muscles and ligaments around a nerve, reducing the amount of pressure and pain that the nerve is under.

In addition, stretching exercises can assist to increase a person's range of motion as well as their flexibility, which further reduces the amount of pressure that is being placed on the nerve. It is important to exercise consistently to achieve optimum outcomes.

However, it is essential to restrain yourself from overdoing it because this might make symptoms worse. Before beginning an exercise routine, those who have been diagnosed with meralgia paresthetica should first speak with a medical professional or a physical therapist.

3. ***Physical therapy***: There is currently no known treatment that will reverse the effects of meralgia paresthetica; however, there are medications that can assist control the symptoms. One example of such a treatment is physical therapy.

   Physical therapists may assist in stretching and strengthening the muscles that are located around the hips, which can help to reduce the pressure that is being placed on the nerve that is being impacted.

   In addition, physical therapists can instruct patients on the most advantageous ways to position their bodies, therefore reducing the likelihood of further compression to the affected area. As a consequence of this, physical therapy has the potential to be an efficient treatment for the management of meralgia paresthetica.

4. ***Stretching***: The pressure and pain associated with the lateral femoral cutaneous nerve can be alleviated by stretching the muscles and ligaments that surround the nerve.

5. ***Massage***: Massage therapy is an excellent treatment for relieving the symptoms of meralgia paresthetica, including pain and numbness in the affected area. In addition, massage therapy can aid in the reduction of inflammation and enhance circulation. As a consequence of this, massage may prove to be an efficient kind of natural treatment for the management of meralgia paresthetica.

6. ***Acupuncture***: A method of treatment utilized in traditional Chinese medicine, acupuncture is characterized by the insertion of very fine needles into specific points on the body. By inducing the release of endorphins, which are the body's naturally occurring painkilling chemicals, acupuncture can be an effective treatment for alleviating pain.

7. ***Herbal Remedies***: Certain herbal treatments might help decrease inflammation and discomfort. Both chamomile and ginger are commonly used for their ability to reduce inflammation, and they may be

consumed either in the form of tea or as capsules. Turmeric, capsaicin, and cayenne pepper are three other botanicals that have potential therapeutic use. Before using any herbal supplements, it is important to discuss the matter with your primary care physician because certain herbal remedies might interfere with other prescriptions.

Meralgia paresthetica is a disorder that has the potential to be both annoying and unpleasant. You can, however, find relief from your symptoms via the use of a variety of natural remedies and treatments. Consuming a balanced diet, engaging in physical activity, and practicing stretching can all contribute to a reduction in pain and inflammation. Alternative treatments such as acupuncture, massage, and herbal medicine may also help relieve symptoms.

Managing Meralgia Paresthetica through Diet

When it comes to the treatment of meralgia paresthetica, diet plays a significant role. It is possible to lessen the severity of symptoms by avoiding items that are known to cause inflammation, such as processed meals, sweets, and unhealthy fats. Consuming foods that are known to lower inflammation, such as those rich in omega-3 fatty acids, may also be beneficial in this regard.

Principles of Meralgia Paresthetica Diet

The principles of a meralgia paresthetica diet are similar to those of an anti-inflammatory diet. This type of diet focuses on reducing inflammation in the body, which can help alleviate symptoms such as pain and discomfort. Here are some key principles to consider when creating a meralgia paresthetica friendly meal plan:

1. **Avoid Processed Foods**

    Highly processed foods often contain high levels of unhealthy fats, sugar, and salt. These ingredients can contribute to increased inflammation in the body and worsen symptoms of meralgia paresthetica, a condition characterized by tingling, numbness, and pain in the outer thigh.

Instead, focus on consuming whole, unprocessed foods such as fresh fruits, colorful vegetables, lean proteins such as chicken and fish, and whole grains like brown rice and quinoa. These nutrient-dense foods provide essential vitamins, minerals, and antioxidants that support overall health and reduce inflammation.

2. Limit Sugar Intake

Excessive sugar consumption can also lead to inflammation in the body, exacerbating conditions like meralgia paresthetica. Sugar can be found in many forms, including sugary drinks, desserts, and processed snacks.

To reduce sugar intake, avoid these high-sugar items and instead opt for natural sweeteners such as honey or maple syrup, which can be used in moderation. Additionally, try incorporating fruits that are naturally sweet, like berries and apples, to satisfy sweet cravings in a healthier way.

3. **Incorporate Omega-3 Fatty Acids**

   Omega-3 fatty acids have well-documented anti-inflammatory properties and can help ease symptoms of meralgia paresthetica by reducing inflammation and promoting nerve health. Some foods that are rich in omega-3s include fatty fish like salmon, mackerel, and tuna, as well as plant-based sources such as chia seeds, flaxseeds, and walnuts.

   Including these foods in your diet can provide the necessary fatty acids to support overall health and potentially alleviate some of the discomfort associated with meralgia paresthetica. Additionally, omega-3 supplements, like fish oil or algae oil, can be considered after consulting with a healthcare provider.

By following these principles, you can create a well-rounded and nutritious diet that may help alleviate symptoms of meralgia paresthetica. It is also important to consult with a healthcare professional or registered dietitian for personalized dietary recommendations based on your individual needs and medical history.

Benefits of a Meralgia Paresthetica Diet

In addition to reducing inflammation, following a meralgia paresthetica diet can also have other benefits for overall health and well-being. Some potential benefits include:

1. ***Weight Management***: Many people with meralgia paresthetica may experience weight gain as a result of decreased physical activity due to pain and discomfort. A healthy, balanced diet can help manage weight and prevent further strain on the affected area, thus alleviating some of the pressure on the nerves. Incorporating nutrient-dense foods such as fruits, vegetables, lean proteins, and whole grains can make a significant difference in maintaining a healthy weight and overall well-being.
2. ***Improved Gut Health***: A diet that is high in whole, unprocessed foods can also promote good gut health by providing essential nutrients and promoting the growth of beneficial gut bacteria. Foods rich in fiber, such as leafy greens, legumes, and whole grains, support digestion and help maintain a healthy gut microbiome. This, in turn, can improve overall health and immunity, which is crucial for managing symptoms and preventing further complications.
3. ***Reduced Risk of Chronic Diseases***: Studies have shown that chronic inflammation in the body can lead to an increased risk of chronic diseases such as heart disease, diabetes, and certain types of cancer. By following a diet that reduces inflammation, such as one rich in omega-3 fatty acids, antioxidants, and phytochemicals found in fruits, vegetables, nuts, and seeds, you may also lower your risk for these

conditions. Reducing processed foods and sugar intake can further help in managing inflammation levels in the body.

4. *Increased Energy Levels*: Eating a well-balanced diet with plenty of fruits, vegetables, and whole grains can provide the necessary nutrients to support energy levels and combat fatigue commonly associated with meralgia paresthetica. Ensuring adequate intake of vitamins and minerals such as B vitamins, iron, and magnesium can support metabolic processes and energy production. Staying hydrated and consuming regular, balanced meals can also help maintain steady energy levels throughout the day, contributing to better overall health and improved quality of life.

Overall, a meralgia paresthetica diet can have a positive impact on both physical and mental well-being, helping individuals manage their symptoms and improve their overall quality of life. However, it is important to remember that each person's dietary needs may vary, so it is crucial to consult with a healthcare professional or registered dietitian for personalized recommendations.

Disadvantages of The Meralgia Paresthetica Diet

Although a meralgia paresthetica diet can offer many potential benefits, there are also some potential drawbacks to consider. Some of these include:

1. **Restrictive Nature**: Depending on the severity of your condition and any underlying health issues, following a specific diet may be quite restrictive and challenging to maintain in the long term. This can lead to feelings of deprivation and make it harder to stick to the dietary guidelines consistently. Additionally, the need to avoid certain foods might limit your dining options, making social outings and gatherings more complicated.
2. **Lack of Convenience**: A meralgia paresthetica diet typically involves preparing meals from scratch using whole, unprocessed foods. This can be time-consuming and may not be feasible for those with busy lifestyles or limited cooking skills. The extra time and effort required for meal planning, grocery shopping, and cooking can be a significant barrier for many people, particularly if they do not enjoy spending time in the kitchen.
3. **Potential Nutrient Deficiencies**: Eliminating certain food groups or following a restrictive diet may lead to nutrient deficiencies if not carefully monitored. It is essential to ensure that you are still consuming a wide

variety of foods to meet your body's nutritional needs. Consulting with a nutritionist or dietitian can help you design a balanced diet plan that avoids deficiencies while still adhering to necessary restrictions.

Despite these potential disadvantages, a meralgia paresthetica diet can still be a helpful tool for managing symptoms and improving quality of life. It is essential to weigh the pros and cons and consult with a healthcare professional before making any significant changes to your diet.

5-Step-by-Step Guide on How to Get Started with Meralgia Paresthetica Diet

When considering implementing a meralgia paresthetica diet, it's essential to have a plan in place. Here is a step-by-step guide on how to get started:

Step 1: Consult Your Healthcare Provider

Begin by scheduling a comprehensive consultation with your healthcare provider or a registered dietitian. During this initial meeting, they will conduct a thorough assessment of your condition, considering factors such as your medical history, current symptoms, and lifestyle habits. This evaluation is crucial because it helps identify any underlying issues that might be contributing to Meralgia Paresthetica.

Your healthcare provider or dietitian will also take into account any other health conditions you may have, ensuring that the dietary recommendations are holistic and safe for you. They can use diagnostic tools, such as blood tests or nutrient deficiency screenings, to gain a better understanding of your overall health status.

Once the assessment is complete, they will provide you with tailored dietary recommendations specifically designed to help manage Meralgia Paresthetica more effectively. These recommendations may include guidelines on portion sizes, meal frequency, and specific foods to emphasize or avoid. They can also suggest supplements if necessary to address any deficiencies or imbalances identified during the consultation.

Additionally, your healthcare provider or dietitian can offer valuable advice on how to integrate these dietary changes into your daily routine seamlessly. They might provide sample meal plans, recipes, and tips for grocery shopping to make the transition easier. Regular follow-up appointments can also be scheduled to monitor your progress, make any necessary adjustments, and ensure that you are on the right track toward managing your condition more effectively.

Step 2: Incorporate Anti-Inflammatory Foods

Incorporating anti-inflammatory foods into your diet is a crucial step in managing Meralgia Paresthetica. These foods can help reduce inflammation and support nerve health, potentially alleviating some of the discomfort associated with the condition.

Here's how you can make these changes effectively:

1. ***Leafy Greens***: Include a variety of leafy greens such as spinach, kale, Swiss chard, and arugula in your meals. These vegetables are rich in vitamins, minerals, and antioxidants that can combat inflammation. You can add them to salads, smoothies, soups, or sauté them as a side dish.
2. ***Fatty Fish***: Fatty fish like salmon, mackerel, sardines, and trout are excellent sources of omega-3 fatty acids, known for their powerful anti-inflammatory properties. Aim to include fatty fish in your diet at least twice a week. You can grill, bake, or poach the fish and pair it with vegetables for a nutritious meal. If fresh fish is not available, consider high-quality canned options or fish oil supplements.
3. ***Nuts and Seeds***: Incorporate nuts such as walnuts, almonds, and seeds like flaxseeds and chia seeds into your diet. These are great sources of healthy fats and antioxidants. You can sprinkle seeds on your yogurt, oatmeal, or salads, and enjoy a handful of nuts as a snack or add them to your dishes for extra crunch and nutrition.
4. ***Fruits***: Focus on consuming anti-inflammatory fruits such as blueberries, strawberries, cherries, and citrus fruits like oranges and grapefruits. These fruits are packed with vitamins, fiber, and antioxidants. Enjoy

them as part of your breakfast, in smoothies, or as a healthy snack throughout the day.
5. **Whole Grains**: Besides the mentioned foods, consider incorporating whole grains like quinoa, brown rice, and oats into your diet. Whole grains contain fiber and other nutrients that support overall health and reduce inflammation.
6. **Herbs and Spices**: Don't forget about herbs and spices such as turmeric, ginger, and garlic, which have potent anti-inflammatory properties. Add these to your cooking for both flavor and health benefits. For instance, turmeric can be added to soups and stews, while ginger can be used in teas and stir-fries.

By systematically incorporating these anti-inflammatory foods into your daily meals, you can create a balanced diet that not only supports nerve health but also enhances your overall well-being. Keep experimenting with different recipes and meal combinations to maintain variety and enjoyment in your diet.

Step 3: Boost Omega-3 Fatty Acids

Increasing your intake of Omega-3 fatty acids is a vital component in managing Meralgia Paresthetica, due to their well-documented anti-inflammatory properties. These essential fats can help reduce inflammation and support nerve health, potentially alleviating the discomfort associated with the condition.

Here's how you can effectively incorporate more Omega-3 fatty acids into your diet:

1. *Flaxseeds*: Flaxseeds are an excellent plant-based source of Omega-3 fatty acids, specifically alpha-linolenic acid (ALA). To reap the benefits, add ground flaxseeds to your smoothies, yogurt, oatmeal, or baked goods. Ground flaxseeds are more easily digestible than whole seeds, maximizing nutrient absorption.
2. *Chia Seeds*: Chia seeds are an excellent source of Omega-3 fatty acids. Their versatility makes them a great addition to many dishes. You can sprinkle them on salads, mix them into your cereal, or make chia pudding by soaking them in almond milk overnight. They also enhance the texture of smoothies and baked goods.
3. *Walnuts*: Walnuts are not only rich in Omega-3 fatty acids but also provide protein and fiber. Enjoy a handful of walnuts as a snack, chop them up to add to salads, or incorporate them into your cooking and baking. Roasted walnuts can enhance the flavor of vegetable dishes and desserts alike.
4. *Fatty Fish*: Fatty fish such as salmon, mackerel, sardines, and trout are among the best sources of

Omega-3s, particularly eicosapentaenoic acid (EPA) and docosahexaenoic acid (DHA). Aim to consume fatty fish at least twice a week. Experiment with different cooking methods like grilling, baking, or poaching to find what you enjoy the most. Pairing fish with nutrient-dense vegetables can make for a balanced meal.

5. *Fish Oil Supplements*: If it's challenging to meet your Omega-3 needs through food alone, consider taking fish oil supplements. Choose high-quality supplements that provide both EPA and DHA. Consult with your healthcare provider before starting any new supplements to ensure they align with your overall health plan and do not interact with other medications.

6. *Other Sources*: Don't overlook other sources of Omega-3s such as hemp seeds, Brussels sprouts, and algae oil. Algae oil is an excellent vegan alternative, offering a direct source of DHA. Incorporate these foods into your diet to diversify your Omega-3 intake.

Practical Tips:

- *Meal Planning*: Plan your meals to include Omega-3-rich foods regularly. For example, add flaxseeds to your breakfast smoothie, enjoy a walnut-studded salad for lunch, and have grilled salmon for dinner.

- ***Recipes***: Try new recipes that highlight Omega-3 ingredients. For instance, make a chia seed pudding for dessert or a walnut-crusted fish fillet for dinner.
- ***Consistency***: Consistency is key. Make these foods a regular part of your diet rather than occasional additions.

By systematically boosting your Omega-3 fatty acid intake, you can support your body's natural anti-inflammatory responses and potentially reduce the symptoms associated with Meralgia Paresthetica. Combining these changes with other dietary adjustments will help create a comprehensive approach to managing your condition.

Step 4: Eliminate Processed and Sugary Foods

Eliminating processed and sugary foods from your diet is a crucial step in managing Meralgia Paresthetica due to its potential to increase inflammation and exacerbate nerve pain. By focusing on whole, natural foods, you can reduce irritation and promote overall better health.

Here's a detailed approach to making this transition:

1. ***Understand the Impact of Processed Foods***: Processed foods often contain high levels of unhealthy fats, refined sugars, and artificial additives. These components can trigger inflammatory responses in the

body. Additionally, they are usually low in essential nutrients, which means they provide empty calories that do not support overall health or nerve function.
2. ***Identify Common Processed Foods***: Start by recognizing the processed foods you regularly consume. This includes items like:
   - Packaged snacks (chips, cookies, crackers)
   - Sugary cereals
   - Fast food
   - Ready-to-eat meals
   - Processed meats (sausages, deli meats, hot dogs)
   - Sweetened beverages (sodas, energy drinks, packaged juices)
3. ***Read Labels***: Develop the habit of reading food labels to identify hidden sugars and artificial ingredients. Look for terms such as high-fructose corn syrup, sucrose, dextrose, and partially hydrogenated oils. Avoid products with long ingredient lists and those containing ingredients you don't recognize.
4. ***Opt for Whole, Natural Foods***: Replace processed and sugary foods with whole, natural alternatives:
   - ***Vegetables***: Fill your plate with a variety of fresh or frozen vegetables. These are packed with vitamins, minerals, and antioxidants that support overall health and help reduce inflammation.

- ***Fruits***: Choose whole fruits instead of fruit juices or sweetened fruit snacks. Berries, apples, oranges, and bananas are nutritious options that make for great snacks or additions to meals.
- ***Whole Grains***: Substitute refined grains with whole grains like quinoa, brown rice, oats, barley, and whole wheat. These provide more fiber and nutrients while helping to maintain stable blood sugar levels.
- ***Lean Proteins***: Include lean sources of protein such as chicken, turkey, tofu, legumes, and fish. These proteins support muscle health and overall body function without contributing to inflammation.
- ***Healthy Fats***: Opt for healthy fats found in avocados, nuts, seeds, and olive oil. These fats support nerve health and have anti-inflammatory properties.

5. ***Healthy Snacking Alternatives***: Swap out sugary snacks for healthier options:
    - Raw veggies with hummus
    - Fresh fruit
    - Plain yogurt with berries
    - Nuts and seeds
    - Whole grain crackers with guacamole

6. *Hydrate Wisely*: Replace sugary beverages with healthier alternatives. Drink water throughout the day to stay hydrated. You can also enjoy herbal teas, infused water with slices of citrus or cucumber, and unsweetened almond milk.
7. *Plan and Prepare Meals*: Planning and preparing your meals can help you avoid processed foods. Cook at home more often, using whole ingredients. Batch cooking and meal prepping can save time and ensure you always have healthy options available.
8. *Mindful Eating*: Practice mindful eating by paying attention to what you eat and how it makes you feel. This can help you make better food choices and recognize the benefits of a cleaner diet.

By eliminating processed and sugary foods and opting for whole, natural alternatives, you can significantly reduce inflammation and manage the symptoms of Meralgia Paresthetica more effectively. This dietary shift will not only help in alleviating nerve pain but also contribute to overall improved health and well-being.

Step 5: Stay Hydrated and Track Your Progress

Staying hydrated and diligently tracking your progress are essential components of managing Meralgia Paresthetica and achieving overall health. Ensuring adequate hydration supports bodily functions and can reduce inflammation, while a food diary helps you identify dietary patterns that impact your symptoms. Here's a detailed guide on how to effectively implement these practices:

1. ***Importance of Hydration***: Water plays a vital role in your body, aiding in digestion, nutrient absorption, and waste elimination. Proper hydration keeps your tissues and joints lubricated and can help maintain nerve health, potentially reducing the discomfort associated with Meralgia Paresthetica. Dehydration, on the other hand, can exacerbate inflammation and aggravate nerve pain.
2. ***Daily Water Intake***: Aim to drink at least 8-10 glasses (about 2-2.5 liters) of water each day. Individual needs can vary based on factors such as activity level, climate, and overall health, so adjust your intake accordingly.

   Strategies to Stay Hydrated:
   - ***Carry a Water Bottle***: Keep a reusable water bottle with you throughout the day to remind yourself to drink regularly.
   - ***Infused Water***: If plain water feels monotonous, try infusing it with slices of lemon, cucumber, mint, or berries for a refreshing twist.
   - ***Set Reminders***: Use smartphone apps or set regular alarms to prompt you to drink water.

- *Eat Water-Rich Foods*: Include foods with high water content in your diet, such as cucumbers, watermelon, strawberries, oranges, and lettuce.

3. *Tracking Your Progress*: Maintaining a food diary is an invaluable tool for managing Meralgia Paresthetica. By documenting what you eat and noting any changes in your symptoms, you can identify which foods may be beneficial or problematic.

    How to Keep a Food Diary:
    - *Daily Entries*: Write down everything you eat and drink each day, including portion sizes and meal times.
    - *Symptom Tracking*: Alongside your food entries, record any symptoms you experience, noting their intensity and duration. This includes pain levels, tingling, numbness, and any other relevant symptoms.
    - *Patterns and Triggers*: Look for patterns over time to identify potential triggers or foods that seem to alleviate your symptoms. For example, you might notice that your pain decreases when you consume more Omega-3-rich foods or increases after eating processed snacks.
    - *Additional Factors*: Include other relevant information such as your physical activity, stress levels, sleep quality, and hydration status.

These factors can also influence your symptoms and provide a more comprehensive picture of your health.

4. ***Regular Review and Adjustments***: Periodically review your food diary and symptom log, ideally every week or two. Share this information with your healthcare provider or dietitian during follow-up appointments. They can help you interpret the data and make informed adjustments to your diet and lifestyle.
5. ***Benefits of Tracking***
   - ***Personalized Insights***: Gain personalized insights into how different foods affect your condition.
   - ***Accountability***: A food diary holds you accountable for your dietary choices and encourages mindful eating.
   - ***Informed Decisions***: Use the data to make informed decisions about which dietary changes are most effective for managing your symptoms.

By staying hydrated and meticulously tracking your dietary intake and symptoms, you can take proactive steps toward managing Meralgia Paresthetica. These practices empower you to optimize your diet, enhance your overall well-being, and work closely with your healthcare provider to make necessary adjustments.

Foods to Eat

When managing Meralgia Paresthetica, it is important to focus on consuming whole, nutrient-dense foods that support overall health and reduce inflammation in the body. Here are some examples of foods you can incorporate into your diet:

1. **Omega-3 Fatty Acid Rich Foods**

   These essential fatty acids are crucial for brain health and reducing inflammation in the body. Foods high in omega-3s include fatty fish such as salmon, sardines, and mackerel. Additionally, plant-based sources like flax seeds, chia seeds, and walnuts are excellent options to incorporate into your diet.

2. **Anti-Inflammatory Spices**

   Spices like turmeric, ginger, and garlic possess potent anti-inflammatory properties that can help reduce swelling and pain in the body. Turmeric contains curcumin, a compound known for its powerful anti-inflammatory effects. Ginger can help alleviate nausea and improve digestion, while garlic is known for boosting the immune system and fighting infections.

3. **Fiber-Rich Foods**

   A diet high in fiber is essential for maintaining good digestive health. Fiber aids in improving digestion, regulating bowel movements, and preventing constipation. Excellent sources of dietary fiber include fruits such as apples, bananas, and berries; vegetables like broccoli, carrots, and leafy greens; legumes such as beans and lentils; whole grains like oats and brown rice; and nuts and seeds.

4. **Colorful Fruits and Vegetables**

Fruits and vegetables that are rich in vibrant colors are packed with antioxidants and essential nutrients that support overall health. These foods can help protect the body from oxidative stress and reduce the risk of chronic diseases. Aiming for a variety of colors in your diet ensures you receive a diverse range of nutrients.

For example, red fruits and vegetables like tomatoes and strawberries are high in lycopene, while orange and yellow options like carrots and sweet potatoes are rich in beta-carotene. Green vegetables such as spinach and kale provide folate and magnesium, while purple and blue options like blueberries and eggplant offer anthocyanins, which have anti-inflammatory effects.

By incorporating these foods into your diet, you can support your body's natural healing processes and promote overall well-being.

Foods to Avoid

Some foods may exacerbate symptoms of Meralgia Paresthetica, so it is important to limit or avoid them in your diet:

- *Processed Foods*: These tend to be high in sugar, unhealthy fats, and preservatives, which can increase inflammation in the body. Consuming a lot of processed foods can lead to various health issues, including weight gain, heart disease, and diabetes. It's advisable to limit your intake of items like packaged snacks, sugary cereals, and fast food.
- *Highly Acidic Foods*: Consuming too many acidic foods (such as citrus fruits, tomatoes, and vinegar) can worsen nerve irritation and potentially lead to acid reflux or other digestive issues. It's best to moderate your intake of these foods and balance them with alkaline foods like leafy greens and other vegetables.
- *Gluten and Dairy Products*: Some people with chronic pain conditions find relief by avoiding gluten and dairy products, as they can cause inflammation and digestive issues in some individuals. Gluten, found in wheat, barley, and rye, can trigger symptoms in those with gluten sensitivity or celiac disease. Dairy, especially full-fat products, can cause discomfort for those who are lactose intolerant or have a dairy allergy.

- ***Highly Refined Carbohydrates***: These include white bread, pasta, and baked goods made with white flour. They have little nutritional value and can contribute to inflammation in the body. Consuming large amounts of these foods can lead to spikes in blood sugar levels and an increased risk of metabolic diseases. Opting for whole grains and fiber-rich alternatives can improve overall health and reduce inflammation.

By reducing or avoiding these foods, you may experience a decrease in symptoms and an improvement in overall health. It is important to listen to your body and make dietary adjustments based on how certain foods make you feel.

Consulting with a healthcare professional or registered dietitian can also be helpful in creating a personalized nutrition plan for managing Meralgia Paresthetica. Remember that every individual's body is unique, so what works for one person may not work for another.

7-Day Sample Meal Plan for Meralgia Paresthetica

To help get you started, here is a sample 7-day meal plan that incorporates some of the foods and nutrients discussed above:

Day 1

Breakfast: Greek yogurt with chia seeds, fresh berries, and a drizzle of honey

Lunch: Fresh Asparagus Salad

Snack: Handful of almonds and an apple

Dinner: Baked Salmon with a side of roasted pumpkin and Brussels sprouts

Day 2

Breakfast: Smoothie with spinach, banana, almond milk, and flaxseeds

Lunch: Tuna Salad

Snack: Carrot sticks with hummus

Dinner: Roasted Chicken Thighs with a side of quinoa stuffed peppers

Day 3

Breakfast: Oatmeal topped with walnuts, blueberries, and a sprinkle of cinnamon

Lunch: Arugula and Mushroom Salad

Snack: Sliced cucumber with guacamole

Dinner: Stir-Fried Cabbage and Apples with a side of baked flounder

Day 4

Breakfast: Scrambled eggs with spinach and tomatoes

Lunch: Asian Zucchini Salad

Snack: Mixed berries

Dinner: Low FODMAP Burger with a side of roasted veggies

Day 5

Breakfast: Quinoa porridge with almond milk, chopped nuts, and dried cranberries

Lunch: Chicken Salad

Snack: Bell pepper slices with tzatziki

Dinner: Roasted Veggies with baked salmon

Day 6

Breakfast: Avocado toast on whole grain bread with a poached egg

Lunch: Asparagus and Greens Salad with Tahini and Poppy Seed Dressing

Snack: Pear slices with a handful of walnuts

Dinner: Roasted Chicken Thighs with stir-fried cabbage and apples

Day 7

Breakfast: Smoothie bowl with mixed berries, almond milk, and granola

Lunch: Asian-Themed Macrobiotic Bowl

Snack: Celery sticks with almond butter

Dinner: Baked Flounder with a side of quinoa stuffed peppers

Sample Recipes

We have included some sample recipes below that incorporate Meralgia Paresthetica-friendly foods and can help provide relief and nourishment to the body:

Baked Flounder

Ingredients:

- 1 lb. flounder, fileted
- 1/4 tsp. salt
- 1 cup halved red grapes
- 1 tbsp. extra-virgin olive oil
- 2 tbsp. parsley, chopped finely
- 1 cup almonds, chopped and toasted
- freshly ground black pepper, to taste

Instructions:

1. Preheat oven to 375°F.
2. Place the flounder filets on a baking sheet lined with parchment paper.
3. Sprinkle salt and pepper over both sides of the filets.
4. In a small bowl, mix together the grapes, olive oil, parsley, almonds, and black pepper.
5. Spoon the mixture onto each filet evenly.
6. Bake for 12-15 minutes or until fish is cooked through and flakes easily with a fork.
7. Serve hot and enjoy!

Asian-Themed Macrobiotic Bowl

Ingredients:

- 2 cups cooked quinoa
- 4 carrots
- 1 package of smoked tofu
- 1 tbsp. nutritional yeast
- 2 tbsp. coconut aminos
- 4 tbsp. sunflower sprouts
- 2 tbsp. fermented vegetables
- 1 cup of shiitake mushrooms
- 1 avocado
- 2 tbsp. hemp seeds
- 2-3 cooked beets
- coconut oil cooking spray

Dressing:

- 2 tbsp. miso paste
- 1 tbsp. tahini
- 1 tbsp. olive oil 3 tbsp. water

Instructions:

1. Preheat the oven to 375°F.
2. Peel and chop carrots into matchsticks.
3. Spray a baking sheet with coconut oil cooking spray and spread out the carrots on it.
4. Bake for 20 minutes, or until tender.

5. Cut tofu into small cubes and marinate in coconut aminos and nutritional yeast for at least 30 minutes.
6. Heat a skillet over medium heat and add marinated tofu, cooking until lightly browned on all sides.
7. In a bowl, layer cooked quinoa, roasted carrots, smoked tofu, sunflower sprouts, fermented vegetables, shiitake mushrooms, sliced avocado and hemp seeds.
8. Whisk together the dressing ingredients in a separate bowl and drizzle over the bowl.
9. Serve and enjoy your delicious Asian-themed macrobiotic bowl!

Chicken Salad

Ingredients:

- 1 small can of premium chunk chicken breast packed in water
- 1 stalk celery, large, finely chopped
- 1/4 cup reduced-fat mayonnaise
- 4 romaine leaves or red leaf lettuce, washed and trimmed
- 1 cucumber, small and sliced thinly

Instructions:

1. Drain the can of chicken and place into a mixing bowl.
2. Using a fork, break apart the chunks of chicken until it is shredded.
3. Add the chopped celery to the chicken and mix together.
4. Measure out 1/4 cup of reduced-fat mayonnaise and add it to the bowl, mixing everything together until well combined.
5. Wash and trim the romaine or red leaf lettuce leaves. Place them on a plate or in a to-go container if you're packing your lunch for work or school.
6. Scoop the chicken salad onto one side of each of your lettuce leaves (about 1/4 cup per lettuce leaf).

7. Roll up each lettuce leaf, starting from the end with the chicken salad and tucking in the sides as you go.
8. Serve with sliced cucumbers on the side or pack them separately for a crunchy addition to your wrap.

Enjoy your delicious and protein-packed chicken salad lettuce wraps!

Baked Salmon

Ingredients:

- 2 salmon filets
- 6 cups of fresh spinach
- 2 tsp. coconut oil
- 1/4 tsp. turmeric
- salt
- pepper

Instructions:

1. Preheat your oven to 400°F (200°C).
2. Place the salmon filets on a baking sheet lined with parchment paper.
3. Rub the coconut oil onto both sides of the salmon filets and season with salt, pepper, and turmeric.
4. Bake in the preheated oven for about 12-15 minutes, until cooked through and flaky.
5. While the salmon is cooking, heat a skillet over medium-high heat and add in the washed spinach along with a pinch of salt and pepper.
6. Cook until the spinach has wilted down, stirring occasionally.

7. Serve the baked salmon on top of a bed of cooked spinach or alongside it for a healthy and nutritious meal packed with omega-3s and leafy greens.

Enjoy your baked salmon with spinach for a quick and easy weeknight meal packed with flavor and nutrients!

Asian Zucchini Salad

Ingredients:

- 1 medium zucchini, sliced thinly into spirals
- 1/3 cup rice vinegar
- 3/4 cup avocado oil
- 1 cup sunflower seeds, shells removed
- 1 lb. cabbage, shredded
- 1 tsp. stevia drops
- 1 cup almonds, sliced

Instructions:

1. In a small bowl, whisk together the rice vinegar, avocado oil, and stevia drops to create the dressing for the salad.
2. In a large mixing bowl, combine the zucchini spirals, shredded cabbage, sunflower seeds, and sliced almonds.
3. Pour the dressing over the salad and toss to evenly coat all ingredients.
4. Serve immediately or store in an airtight container in the fridge for up to 3 days.

This Asian zucchini salad is perfect as a side dish or add some protein like grilled chicken or tofu for a complete meal option.

Enjoy this refreshing and healthy salad as part of your daily vegetable intake!

Low FODMAP Burger

Ingredients:

- 1-1/4 lbs. ground pork
- 1/2 tsp. salt
- 1/2 tsp. white pepper
- 1/2 tsp. ground nutmeg
- 1/2 tsp. caraway seeds
- 1/2 tsp. ground ginger

Instructions:

1. In a large mixing bowl, combine the ground pork and all spices.
2. Mix well until all ingredients are evenly incorporated into the meat.
3. Form the mixture into 4 equal-sized patties.
4. Heat a grill or grill pan to medium-high heat and lightly oil the surface.
5. Place the burger patties on the heated surface and cook for 5-6 minutes on each side, or until fully cooked through.
6. Serve on your choice of gluten-free bun or lettuce wrap with your favorite toppings such as lettuce, tomato, and avocado.

This low-FODMAP burger is perfect for those following a low-FODMAP diet due to digestive sensitivities or IBS.

Enjoy this tasty and gut-friendly burger as a satisfying meal option!

Asparagus and Greens Salad with Tahini and Poppy Seed Dressing

Ingredients:

- 10 to 12 asparagus stalks, washed well and sliced into ribbons
- 5 radishes, washed well and sliced thinly
- 2 to 3 rainbow carrots, peeled and sliced thinly
- 1 handful of wild spinach
- 1 small handful of microgreens, washed well
- 1 small handful of sunflower greens, washed well
- optional: a few pieces of chive blossoms

For the dressing:

- 2 tbsp. tahini
- 1 tbsp. poppy seeds
- 1 tbsp. extra-virgin olive oil
- salt
- pepper

Instructions:

1. In a large mixing bowl, combine the sliced asparagus, radishes, and carrots.
2. Add in the wild spinach, microgreens, and sunflower greens.
3. Toss everything together until well mixed.

4. In a separate small mixing bowl, whisk together the tahini, poppy seeds, olive oil, salt, and pepper to make the dressing.
5. Drizzle the dressing over the salad mixture and toss to coat evenly.
6. Optional: sprinkle with chive blossoms for added flavor and presentation.
7. Serve as a refreshing and nutritious lunch option or as a side dish for dinner.

Stir-Fried Cabbage and Apples

Ingredients:

- 1 shallot, thinly sliced
- 1/2 apple, cut into cubes
- 1/4 savoy cabbage, sliced thinly into strips
- 3–4 radishes, sliced thinly
- 1/2–1 tsp. coconut oil
- salt, to taste

Instructions:

1. In a large pan or wok, heat the coconut oil over medium-high heat.
2. Add in the shallot and cook until softened about 2 minutes.
3. Stir in the cubed apples and continue cooking for another minute.
4. Add in the sliced cabbage and radishes, stirring constantly to mix everything together.
5. Cook for about 5-7 minutes, until the cabbage is slightly wilted but still has some crunch.
6. Season with salt to taste.
7. Serve as a side dish or add protein like seared tofu or grilled shrimp for a complete meal option.

This stir-fried cabbage and apple dish is also great as leftovers, making it an ideal meal prep option for busy weekdays!

Roasted Chicken Thighs

Ingredients:

- 1 tbsp. avocado oil
- 1 pinch Himalayan pink salt
- 4 chicken thighs with skin
- 1 tsp. Primal Palate super gyro seasoning

Instructions:

1. Preheat the oven to 375°F (190°C).
2. In a large mixing bowl, toss the chicken thighs with avocado oil and Himalayan pink salt.
3. Sprinkle super gyro seasoning over the chicken thighs, coating both sides evenly.
4. Place chicken thighs on a baking sheet lined with parchment paper or aluminum foil.
5. Roast in the oven for about 30 minutes, until golden brown and crispy on the outside and cooked through on the inside.
6. Serve hot as a main dish with your favorite side dishes like roasted vegetables or a salad.
7. Leftover chicken can be stored in an airtight container in the fridge for up to 3 days for easy meal prep options throughout the week.

Arugula and Mushroom Salad

Ingredients:

- 5 oz. arugula washed
- 1 lb. fresh mushrooms
- 1/4 tsp. shoyu
- 1 tbsp. olive oil
- 1 tbsp. mirin

For tofu cheese:

- 1/8 cup umeboshi vinegar
- 1/2 firm tofu

Instructions:

1. Wash and dry arugula and place in a large mixing bowl.
2. Slice mushrooms thinly and add to the bowl with arugula.
3. In a small mixing bowl, whisk together shoyu, olive oil, and mirin to make dressing.
4. Pour dressing over the arugula and mushroom mixture, tossing well to coat evenly.

5. For the tofu cheese: In a separate small mixing bowl, mash firm tofu with umeboshi vinegar until it forms a creamy consistency.
6. Toss the tofu cheese into the salad and mix well.
7. Serve as a refreshing side dish or add protein like grilled chicken or shrimp for a complete meal option.

Fresh Asparagus Salad

Ingredients:

- 1/3 cup of hazelnuts
- 4 cups arugula
- 1 tsp. ground pepper
- 2 tbsp. sea salt
- virgin olive oil
- 2 lbs. asparagus

Instructions:

1. Preheat the oven to 400°F.
2. Place hazelnuts on a baking tray with parchment paper. Place in the oven for 7 minutes.
3. Transfer hazelnuts to a plate. Optionally, to remove the skins, wrap the nuts in a towel and rub them vigorously.
4. Chop hazelnuts coarsely.
5. Remove the hard ends of the asparagus.
6. Place the stalks on the baking sheet you've used for the hazelnuts. Sprinkle 1 tbsp. olive oil and 1/2 tsp. of salt.
7. Bake for 8 minutes.
8. In a mixing bowl, combine pepper, salt, and olive oil. Mix well.

9. Place the arugula in a medium bowl. Drizzle half of the dressing over the veggies. Toss until everything is well coated.
10. Place arugula onto a platter.
11. Arrange asparagus on top. Sprinkle peeled hazelnuts on top.

Tuna Salad

Ingredients:

- 1/2 cup pecans
- 1 cup chicken breast, steamed and cubed
- 1 cup tuna in oil
- salt, to taste
- pepper, to taste

Instructions:

1. Preheat the oven to 350°F.
2. Spread pecans on a baking tray with parchment paper. Place in the oven for 5-7 minutes until fragrant and lightly toasted.
3. Remove from oven and let cool for a few minutes before chopping them coarsely.
4. In a mixing bowl, combine chicken breast, tuna, salt, and pepper.
5. Add chopped pecans to the mixture.
6. Mix well until all ingredients are evenly distributed.
7. Serve as a sandwich filling or over a bed of greens for a hearty salad option.

Roasted Veggies

Ingredients:

- 1/2 lb. turnips
- 1/2 lb. carrots
- 1/2 lb. parsnips
- 2 shallots, peeled
- 1/4 tsp. ground black pepper
- 1 tbsps. extra-virgin olive oil
- 6 cloves of garlic
- 3/4 tsp. kosher salt
- 2 tbsp. fresh rosemary needles

Instructions:

1. Preheat oven to 400°F.
2. Peel and cut turnips, carrots, and parsnips into bite-sized chunks.
3. Place the veggies in a large bowl.
4. Add shallots, rosemary needles, pepper, salt, and garlic cloves to the bowl.
5. Drizzle olive oil over the vegetables and mix well until everything is evenly coated.
6. Spread the vegetable mixture onto a baking sheet lined with parchment paper.

7. Bake for 30-35 minutes or until vegetables are soft and slightly caramelized on the edges.
8. Serve as a side dish or add to your favorite salad for an extra boost of flavor and nutrients.

Roasted Pumpkin and Brussels Sprouts

Ingredients:

- 3 lb. pie pumpkin, peeled and cut into ¾-inch cubes
- 1 lb. fresh Brussels sprouts, trimmed and halved lengthwise
- 1 tsp. sea salt
- 1/2 tsp. coarsely ground pepper
- 1/3 cup olive oil
- 2 tbsp. balsamic vinegar
- 2 tbsp. minced fresh parsley
- 4 garlic cloves, thinly sliced

Instructions:

1. Preheat oven to 400°F.
2. In a large mixing bowl, toss pumpkin cubes and Brussels sprouts with salt, pepper, olive oil, balsamic vinegar, parsley, and garlic slices.
3. Spread the mixture onto a baking sheet lined with parchment paper.
4. Roast for 30-35 minutes or until vegetables are tender and lightly browned.
5. Serve as a side dish or add to your favorite grain bowl for a delicious and filling meal option.

Quinoa Stuffed Peppers

Ingredients:

- 4 sweet bell peppers, halved vertically, with ribs and seeds removed
- 3/4 cup quinoa, well rinsed
- 15 oz. tomatoes, diced
- 4 cups basil leaves
- 10 oz. baby spinach
- 1 clove of garlic, small
- 1/4 cup pistachios, unsalted
- 6 tbsp. grated parmesan cheese
- 3 tbsp. extra-virgin olive oil
- 3 tbsp. boiling water
- 1/4 tsp. kosher salt
- a pinch of black pepper, freshly ground

Instructions:

1. Combine the basil, garlic, parmesan cheese, olive oil, black pepper, and a pinch of salt in a food processor or blender.
2. Blend until the texture of the mixture appears finely chopped.
3. Stir in the boiling water.

To make the stuffed peppers:

1. Place the bell pepper halves with the side up on a lightly oiled baking sheet.
2. Roast in the oven using the high setting for about 10 minutes, or until they start to soften and have become slightly charred.
3. Remove the peppers from the oven. Set them aside.
4. In a medium pot, let the quinoa and tomatoes simmer in the vegetable broth for 10 minutes.
5. Stir in the baby spinach in small batches.
6. Scoop the quinoa-spinach mixture. Place them into the roasted peppers.
7. Drizzle the filled bell peppers with pesto sauce.
8. Garnish with pistachios on top upon serving.

Conclusion

As you reach the end of this guide on managing meralgia paresthetica through diet, it's essential to reflect on the considerable impact that nutrition can have on your condition. Diet is more than just a collection of foods; it's a powerful ally in your journey to alleviate the discomfort and symptoms associated with this nerve disorder.

Meralgia paresthetica, characterized by tingling, numbness, and burning pain in the outer thigh, can significantly affect your quality of life. However, adjusting your diet can be a transformative step toward managing these symptoms. Throughout this guide, we have delved into how certain foods can reduce inflammation, support nerve health, and contribute to overall well-being.

Incorporating anti-inflammatory foods into your daily meals is one of the key strategies discussed. Foods rich in omega-3 fatty acids, such as salmon, chia seeds, and walnuts, are known for their anti-inflammatory properties. These foods can help reduce the nerve inflammation that contributes to the discomfort of meralgia paresthetica. Similarly, a diet abundant in fruits and vegetables, particularly those high in antioxidants like berries, spinach, and bell peppers, can protect your nerves from oxidative stress and aid in their repair.

Another critical aspect highlighted is the importance of vitamins and minerals. Vitamin B12, found in animal products like meat, fish, and dairy, is crucial for nerve function and repair. A deficiency in this vitamin can exacerbate the symptoms of meralgia paresthetica. Additionally, magnesium, which is present in foods like nuts, seeds, and whole grains, plays a vital role in muscle and nerve function. Ensuring that your diet includes these essential nutrients can make a significant difference in managing your symptoms.

Maintaining a healthy weight is another vital component of managing meralgia paresthetica through diet. Excess body weight can exert additional pressure on your nerves, worsening the symptoms. Adopting a balanced diet that emphasizes whole grains, lean proteins, and healthy fats can not only help you manage your weight but also provide sustained energy and reduce inflammation.

Hydration is an often overlooked aspect of dietary management. Staying adequately hydrated helps maintain optimal body function and can reduce the sensation of pain. Drinking plenty of water and avoiding excessive consumption of dehydrating beverages like caffeine and alcohol can support your overall health and help manage your symptoms more effectively.

As you move forward, it's important to remember that diet alone may not fully resolve the symptoms of meralgia paresthetica. Integrating other lifestyle changes, such as regular physical activity tailored to your condition, ergonomic adjustments in your daily routine, and stress management techniques, will create a more holistic approach to managing your health. Consulting with healthcare providers, including nutritionists and physical therapists, can provide you with a personalized plan that addresses all aspects of your health.

Creating sustainable dietary habits is about making gradual, manageable changes rather than drastic overhauls. Listening to your body and observing how it responds to different foods will guide you in fine-tuning your diet to best suit your needs. The goal is to establish a lifestyle that supports your long-term health and alleviates the symptoms of meralgia paresthetica.

Engaging with supportive communities, whether online or in person, can be incredibly beneficial. Sharing experiences, recipes, and tips with others who understand what you're going through can provide additional motivation and emotional support. It also helps to stay informed about the latest research and developments in nutritional science related to nerve health.

Your commitment to learning about and implementing these dietary strategies is commendable. By taking an active role in managing your health, you are empowering yourself to live a more comfortable and fulfilling life despite the challenges of meralgia paresthetica. Every small step you take towards better nutrition and overall well-being is a victory worth celebrating.

Thank you for dedicating your time and attention to reading this comprehensive guide on managing meralgia paresthetica through diet. Your willingness to educate yourself and make informed decisions about your health is truly inspiring. Remember, the journey to better health is ongoing, and every positive change you make, no matter how small, contributes to your overall progress.

FAQs

What is meralgia paresthetica?

Meralgia paresthetica is marked by tingling, numbness, and a burning sensation in the outer thigh. This condition arises when the lateral femoral cutaneous nerve becomes compressed or injured, which can be caused by wearing tight clothing, being overweight, or standing for extended periods.

Can diet really help manage meralgia paresthetica symptoms?

Yes, diet can play a significant role in managing the symptoms of meralgia paresthetica. A diet rich in anti-inflammatory foods, vitamins, and minerals can help reduce nerve inflammation, support nerve health, and promote overall well-being, potentially alleviating some of the discomfort associated with the condition.

Which foods should I include in my diet to help with meralgia paresthetica?

Incorporating foods high in omega-3 fatty acids like salmon, walnuts, and flaxseeds can reduce inflammation.

Antioxidant-rich fruits and vegetables such as berries, spinach, and bell peppers protect nerves from oxidative stress. Additionally, foods rich in vitamin B12 (meat, fish, dairy) and magnesium (nuts, seeds, whole grains) support nerve function and repair.

Are there any foods I should avoid to prevent worsening my symptoms?

It's advisable to limit the intake of processed foods, sugars, and trans fats, as these can increase inflammation and potentially worsen symptoms. Reducing the consumption of alcohol and caffeine, which can dehydrate and affect nerve health, may also be beneficial.

How does maintaining a healthy weight impact meralgia paresthetica?

Maintaining a healthy weight is crucial because excess body weight can place additional pressure on the nerves, exacerbating the symptoms of meralgia paresthetica. Adopting a balanced diet that helps manage weight can reduce this pressure and alleviate discomfort.

Is hydration important in managing meralgia paresthetica symptoms?

Yes, staying adequately hydrated is important for overall health and can help manage the symptoms of meralgia paresthetica. Proper hydration supports optimal body function and can reduce pain perception. Drinking plenty of water and limiting dehydrating beverages like caffeine and alcohol is recommended.

Should I consult with healthcare professionals about my diet for managing meralgia paresthetica?

Consulting with healthcare providers, including nutritionists and physical therapists, can provide you with a personalized plan tailored to your specific needs. They can help ensure that your dietary choices effectively support your condition and overall health.

References and Helpful Links

How do you treat meralgia paresthetica? Symptoms & causes. (2020, June 12). eMedicineHealth. https://www.emedicinehealth.com/how_do_you_treat_meralgia_paresthetica/article_em.htm

Meralgia paresthetica - what you need to know. (n.d.). Drugs.com. https://www.drugs.com/cg/meralgia-paresthetica.html

Prakash, J. (2017, June 20). Meralgia paresthetica: treatment, diet and home remedies. mTatva Health-PIE. https://www.mtatva.com/en/disease/meralgia-paresthetica-treatment-diet-and-home-remedies/

Meralgia paresthetica - Diagnosis and treatment - Mayo Clinic. (2024, January 26). https://www.mayoclinic.org/diseases-conditions/meralgia-paresthetica/diagnosis-treatment/drc-20355639

Sekul, E. A., MD. (n.d.). Meralgia paresthetica: background, pathophysiology, epidemiology. https://emedicine.medscape.com/article/1141848-overview

Meralgia paresthetica. (2020, March 27). Johns Hopkins Medicine. https://www.hopkinsmedicine.org/health/conditions-and-diseases/meralgia-paresthetica#:~:text=Meralgia%20Paresthetica%20Treatment&text=Ph

ysical%20therapy%20to%20strengthen%20the,Corticosteroid%20injecti on%20to%20reduce%20swelling

Meralgia Paresthetica: a beginner's quick start guide to managing the condition through diet and other home remedies, with sample curated recipes: Marshwell, Patrick: 9798849629971: Amazon.com: Books. (n.d.).
https://www.amazon.com/Meralgia-Paresthetica-Beginners-Managing-Condition/dp/B0BCSB1GGG

Brain Center. (2022, November 18). Foods to Avoid or Incorporate When Living with Neuropathy.
https://braincenter.org/2022/11/18/foods-to-avoid-or-incorporate-when-living-with-neuropathy/#:~:text=Foods%20to%20Avoid%3A,and%20can%20worsen%20neuropathy%20symptoms.

www.ingramcontent.com/pod-product-compliance
Lightning Source LLC
LaVergne TN
LVHW012034060526
838201LV00061B/4597